The U.S. Constitution

The Articles of Confederation are one of the most cherished documents in American history. They have been reduced to a footnote. Americans tend to overlook the time period between 1783, when peace was reached, and 1787, when the Constitution was drafted. To understand the Constitution, you must first understand its origins.

The new United States tried to operate after the Revolution under the Articles of Confederation. These Articles had been written in wartime by men who were concerned about Parliamentary abuses of power. It is not surprising, then, that the national government that the Continental Congress created during the Revolutionary War was weak.

The reason Congress couldn't pay soldiers in the war was because Congress was unable to pay them during the actual war.

The Continental Army was not able to tax because it did no have the power. The Continental Congress was constantly pestered by General George Washington for provisions, but could only request money from the States.

Because Parliament had abused its authority against colonies, the Articles of Confederation were deliberately avoided by the drafters. However, it wasn't long before this became a serious limitation on the national government. The inability of the national governments to raise revenue also made foreign policy difficult. The United States was without a navy after the Revolutionary War and no longer had protection from the British navy.

The result was that American commerce was taken by Barbary pirates. However, Congress couldn't do anything to stop them because it couldn't raise enough money to finance a navy to protect American shipping.

The Articles of Confederation also made it impossible for the Congress to pay any debts it had incurred to foreign powers in the Revolutionary War. Even though the allied powers had loaned the American government at favorable terms, and no repayment was expected before the end of hostilities ended, there was little chance of the Congress ever being able to pay its national debts without a tax-paying national government. The

Articles of Confederation were ended because of the possibility of the new nation defaulting upon its French loans.

The Articles of Confederation did not have an executive or judiciary branch. The Congress passed laws, but they could not be implemented by the national government. This left the enforcement of laws to the state. The same goes for national law disputes.

It was evident that the Articles of Confederation did not suit the needs of the new nation by 1787. These problems hampered the national government's ability to function under the Articles of Confederation. With the threat of defaulting on the nation's huge war debt, plans were made to address the Articles of Confederation. In the summer of 1876, a Constitutional Convention was called and all states sent delegates to Philadelphia. Some of the delegates included prominent patriots, former members of Continental Congress, and Benjamin Franklin.

While most delegates arrived to Philadelphia with little, Alexander Hamilton, James Madison, and others were well-prepared and had studied extensively. Hamilton was a pioneer in calling for a Constitutional Convention in order to restructure our nation's government. He had also been an advocate at Annapolis' convention a year before. Hamilton was elected to write a document explaining the reasons for a stronger nation's government at that convention. It was sent to each state and was instrumental in bringing about the Constitutional Convention opening in 1787.

Madison was also working on his political theory, and had prepared extensively for the Convention. Madison utilized his vast knowledge of foreign and ancient languages to study Constitutions across the globe. This was something he had done before helping to craft the Virginia Constitution. He was an authority on Constitutionalism. Because of his background and the fact that he was a better researcher than anyone else at the Convention, the Convention delegates considered him a leader in the field.

The Constitutional Convention was held in Philadelphia on May 14, 1787. Madison was not only the first to arrive, but he also had a plan for a national government. Because it was supported by Virginia's delegation (of which Madison was part), this plan was known as the Virginia Plan. Most of the other delegates arrived in Philadelphia empty-handed and had not even opened a single book about the topic. This was due to the fact the Philadelphia Convention's original intent wasn't to create a new government, but to reform it. Madison arrived in Philadelphia carrying a plan, the Virginia Plan. He quickly distributed it to the other delegates, before proceedings even started.

Hamilton, who had made loud calls for stronger national governments and helped to establish the Convention, was pushed aside.

Madison. Hamilton was naturally a delegate at the Constitutional

Convention. However, it was surprising that his louder calls for stronger national governments became less vocal at the Convention. Hamilton felt intellectually inferior and marginalized at the Convention, but this was not because of his new views. Hamilton was also supported by his fellow New York Representatives, but Hamilton felt marginalized and inferior at the Convention. Since states vote as units, Hamilton's view was not represented in his own delegation.

Madison didn't introduce the Virginia Plan. Instead, Virginia Governor Edmund Randolph presented the plan to the Convention. Delegates implicitly voted for a complete overhaul of Articles of Confederation when they voted whether to vote. The Virginia plan was so distinct from the Articles that the Convention voted to consider it. The Convention voted almost unanimously to create a new Constitution and the debate began.

While the U.S. Constitution made some significant departures from Madison's Virginia Plan, Madison's work was the blueprint. Madison's Plan called to have a bicameral legislature with each chamber made up of representatives from each state. This would be proportional to each state's population. This was favorable for large states such as Virginia, which at the time was the most populous. The Virginia Plan, over the course the convention, became the Big State Plan. Madison's Plan made a lasting contribution by establishing the terms for the separation of power and a three-branch government consisting of legislative, judiciary, and executive branches. Each branch was to be distinct from the others, and each would have different powers and functions that allowed them to "check" the power in the other branches. This was a radical departure from other forms, such as the English Parliamentarian System, in which the Prime Minister was simultaneously a member of both the legislative and executive branches of government.

Although the structure of the three branches was generally agreed upon, there was much disagreement over how the two houses of national legislature were allocated. Madison's Big State Plan was quickly rejected by smaller states, and they voted for the New Jersey Plan with some modifications. This plan provided for equal representation in all states through a unicameral legislature. Although most of the New Jersey Plan was never seriously considered, the idea that all states should be equal represented made it into the Constitution's formula to elect the U.S. Senate. Madison opposed the plan, arguing the smaller states should not be worried about being overthrown by the larger. Madison and Hamilton argued together that the large states like New York, Massachusetts and Pennsylvania were so different from one another that they could not form an alliance that would dominate the national government at cost of small states. Other states could also ally with large ones, making the argument of large state dominance moot. The New England states would support Massachusetts, while the Southern states would consider Virginia to be the leader. Meanwhile, the mid-Atlantic would divide between Pennsylvania and New York.

The Constitution marked a departure from the Articles of Confederation, which were criticized by the Constitution's proponents as promoting dissonance and too much autonomy for the States. They believed that a strong federal government should be able to provide for a national army, maintain standing armies, and levy direct taxes to help its common defense and promote economic prosperity. [1] Some people are concerned about the federal government becoming too powerful and abusing its tax or military authority. They suggest that they should understand the role of the legislature or representatives of the people in determining whether the central government has the authority to raise an army or levy taxes. This was a new democratic experiment, one that had never been attempted before. [2]

There are many reasons why the final draft of Constitution, which was approved by the Committee of Style on September 12, and embossed on October 15th, didn't include a list of enumerated right. The men proposing different plans for the Constitution did not have a complete list, despite the heat in the room.

You can find the reason in most history textbooks. John Locke's natural rights ("life liberty, property") were granted to any government by any government since the Declaration of Independence explicitly states that they were given to people when they were born. This is perhaps the reason Madison's Virginia Plan was not approved by Paterson's New Jersey Plan. It was also the reason why Paterson's New Jersey Plan was not approved. The Bill of Rights in Virginia was the most well-known, but many other states had already enumerated rights so it was assumed that the national government wouldn't need one. This would need to be addressed as Madison and Hamilton tried to convince the states to ratify it.

However, this does not mean that Constitution writers did not include certain rights. They included the rights they felt most strongly about in the Constitution, mainly the rights that govern a nation's legal spheres. Ex post facto laws, which make acts punishable later in the case, bills of attainder (which makes laws to aid or discriminate against individuals) and suspension of habeas corpus other than during rebellion are all prohibited by the Constitution. These were all based on experiences during the 1760s & 1770s.

Mason was present at the Virginia delegates meeting to propose that a bill be added after the Committee of Style had returned with its draft. It was not. [3]

Nearly all the delegates present signed the document on September 17. (Interestingly, Rhode Island did not send any and New York's was recalled with Hamilton as exception). Elbridge Gerry, George Mason and Edmund Randolph were the only remaining delegates to refuse to sign the new Constitution. However, given the absence of delegates from Philadelphia on September 17, less that 40 delegates signed the document.

Although Madison did not get all he desired from the Constitution that was ultimately drafted, no one else did. Benjamin Franklin delivered a speech on the day that the Constitution was signed. It summarised many of the thoughts of the delegate and explained why he would vote for it. As I get older, my judgments are more suspect and I pay more attention to others' judgments. Sir, these sentiments sum up why I support this Constitution. I believe a general Government is necessary for us. I also believe that there is no other form of Government than what may be a blessing for the people if it is well administered. I further believe that this will only end in Despotism when the people will become corrupt enough to require despotic government. I also doubt that any other Convention, which we may obtain, could be better at making a Constitution. You can't assemble many men without having the benefit of their collective wisdom. Therefore, you will undoubtedly assemble with them, all their prejudices and passions, as well as their errors of mind, local interests, and selfish views. A perfect production can only be expected from such an assembly. It is therefore surprising to me Sir that this system comes so close to perfection. I believe it will also astonish our enemies who are eager to hear that our Councils are confused like the Builders at Babel and that our States are about to split, with the sole purpose of cutting each other's throats. Sir, I agree to this Constitution, because I don't expect anything better and because it isn't the best. I will sacrifice my opinions about its mistakes for the greater good of the public. I have never spoken a word of them outside. They were born within these walls, and they will die here."

The U.S. Constitution would still need to be ratified and ratified by the States. They would then have to ratify it according to the guidelines set out in the original Articles. This stipulated that at least 9 of the 13 states had to agree to it. "The ratification by nine states of the conventions shall be sufficient to establish this Constitution between those states that have ratified the same."[4]

Madison saw this coming and used the opportunity to reward individual delegate by using their input during the drafting of the Constitution. This would provide them with all the incentive they needed to ratify it. "Madison already had the key insight into unorthodox legitimation. He was not aiming for one grand victory but rather a stepwise process where each partial initiative builds on the previous in a series sequential ratifications."[5]

Madison said, "The attempts to bring about a correction through the medium of Congress have failed." Let us then try a Convention. If the Convention succeeds in its first instance, other defects will be brought to the public's attention and the public will be prepared for more remedies. The Assembly [in Virginia] would not refer to Congress. They would have rebelled equally against the plenipotentiary Commission to their deputies in the Convention. There was only one option: do what was done or do nothing. It is impossible to prove whether a right decision was made in the end. I'm not a proponent of partial or temporizing remedies. However, too much rigor in this regard can lead to everything." [6]

It would still require a lot of work, despite everyone's efforts. There were many public discussions between supporters and opponents of the new Constitution, which took place from October 1787 to August 1788. The question was whether the United States would continue to be governed by Articles of Confederation, or adopt the new Constitution. The Articles of Confederation today are considered an archaic failure. However, it is important to recall that the Constitution required 13 states to give up substantial amounts of their sovereignty in order to ratify it.

The Constitution is today a sacred document in the United States. However, there was much debate about whether or not it should be ratified. Federalists were the name given to those who voted for the new Constitution, in reference to the new federalism it embodied. Opponents were called Anti-Federalists.

Many Anti-Federalists were concerned about the new

The Constitution created a stronger national government with a strong executive and a vague judiciary, but it did not include a Bill of Rights that would protect citizens from these new entities. Many state Constitutions included bills of rights that protected citizens from the state's power. The Bill of Rights in England was one of the most important Constitutional documents. The Bill of Rights supporters had attempted to amend the Constitution before its adoption but failed. Many believed that it was dangerous to adopt a new Constitution without having a bill in place.

Leading Federalists and Anti-Federalists authored essays shortly after the Convention arguing in favor or against the adoption and responding to arguments from the opposing side. Hamilton, despite his initial objections to the Convention, was a pragmaticist and believed that the Constitution proposed was a strong compromise. While it preserved some state sovereignty, it significantly increased the power of federal government. He advocated that all states ratify this new document. Hamilton was the one who sold the Constitution to the American people. He recruited James Madison and John Jay, and they wrote anonymously a series of letters in support of the Constitution. These writings became collectively known as the Federalist Papers. They are still cited regularly by jurists and politicians in America today.

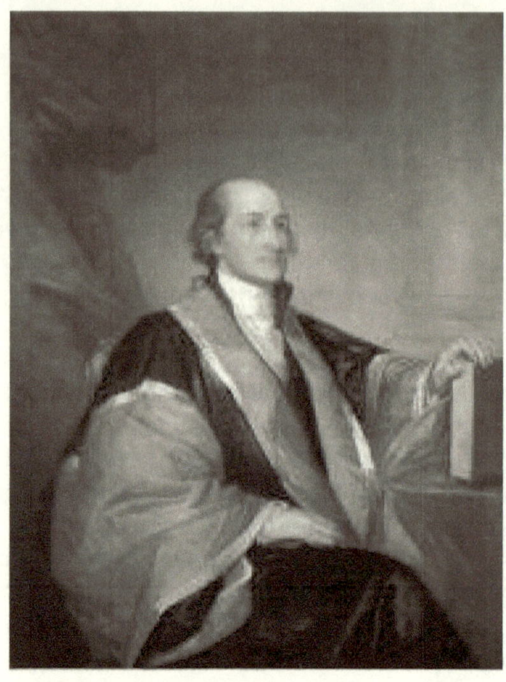

Jay

Hamilton was the author of most of the Federalist Papers. However, all papers were signed under the pseudonym of "Publius." Hamilton's most important pieces are about the principle of judicial reviewing. Madison's writings are the most influential and still being read today. These include the Federalist #10, Federalist #51 and other notable pieces. Madison did not write as much about the Federalist Papers as Hamilton, but the Virginian is remembered as the "Father" of the Constitution and the most articulate advocate for it.

Although they are well-known today, the Federalist Papers played a smaller role in the debate about ratification. Their popularity has only increased due to the fact that they were almost entirely written by Madison and Hamilton. The Federalist Papers were rarely reprinted beyond New York. Some historians claim that they were intended more as a guidebook for ratification proponents to use when arguing in support of the Constitution.

The Federalist Papers continue to be of great importance to Constitutional law scholars, lawyers, and judges. The Federalist Papers are not only important, but they also have a significant impact on the lives of judges and lawyers.

While Federalist Papers can still be used to determine the intent of the Founding Generation, not all Founding members gave them much respect. McCulloch v. Maryland was the case that established the supremacy and control of federal law over state laws. Chief Justice John Marshall observed that the Federalist Papers were "justly assumed to be entitled to high respect in expounding on the Constitution." They deserve no tribute that exceeds their merit. However, in applying their opinions in the context of the government's progress, it is important to retain the right to determine their accuracy. Marshall, America's greatest justice, privately stated that "the legitimate meaning" of the Instrument must come from the text. If a key is needed elsewhere, it must not be in the intentions or opinions of the Body which proposed it, but the sense given to it by the people at their State Conventions. All the authority it has."

Federalist Papers recognized that only a few words on parchment might be enough. Federalist No. 59 stated it very prophetically by Hamilton. 59: "If we are in a comedy to presume abuses, it is as fair as to presume them on behalf of the State governments as the general government."

Madison was a strong advocate for ratifying the Constitution. However, he was also acutely aware of its critics' opinions. Madison suggested that the new Constitution be attached with a Bill of Rights that would clearly define individuals' rights. Hamilton opposed the idea, believing that it was unnecessary and that explicit listing certain rights might imply that governments would have any rights not specifically listed. The Bill of Rights was a resounding defeat for central government.

Contrary to Hamilton's argument Madison's main concern about a Bill of Rights would be that it would open up the door for further debate on the merits of Constitution. This could lead to the collapse of the whole system. Madison stated in a 1789 speech before Congress that he was not willing to see a way opened to re-examine the entire structure of government and to re-examine the substance and principles of the powers granted. Because I doubt that if such a door were opened, it would make it very unlikely for us to stop at the point which would be safe for the government.

Madison was the one who first created the Bill of Rights. Madison suggested about 20 possible Amendments. However, the original Bill of Rights contained 10 Amendments. These are central to American freedoms. They include the 1st Amendment's freedom of expression, the 4th Amendment ban on illegal search or seizure, and the 5th Amendments' Due Process. Also, criminal defense and civil trial rights are guaranteed by the 5th-6th, 7th, and 8th Amendments. Hamilton's main concern was addressed by the 10th Amendment. It reserved all powers that were not specifically listed in the Constitution for the people.

States are reserved for the States or the people.

The new structure of the national government meant that the president position had to be filled. One man was chosen for the position. The delegates unanimously agreed that Washington was the best chief executive for the new country. They had created the office of president with Washington's ideas in mind.

Washington provided a rare glimpse into his thoughts during his inauguration. There's no doubt that Washington was thinking about some of the Philadelphia debates from 1787. Washington spoke out against the "local prejudices and attachments" of 13 states. He also warned about "separate opinions or animosities.".

Washington stated that the debated area of republicanism, freedom and liberty, was not the only one. He said to his audience that the foundation of our national policies would be the simple and unalterable principles of private morality. The preeminence and primacy of free government will be demonstrated by all attributes that can win the admiration of its citizens and earn the respect of the rest of the world.

In a 1790 letter to an acquaintance, Vice President John Adams stated that he dreaded the division of the republic into two great political parties, each one arranged under its leader and taking concerted measures against each other. This is, in my humble apprehension to be the most serious political evil under our Constitution."

   Alexander Hamilton, Secretary of Treasury, and Thomas Jefferson, Secretary of State were involved in the debates that would lead to the creation of the first political parties.

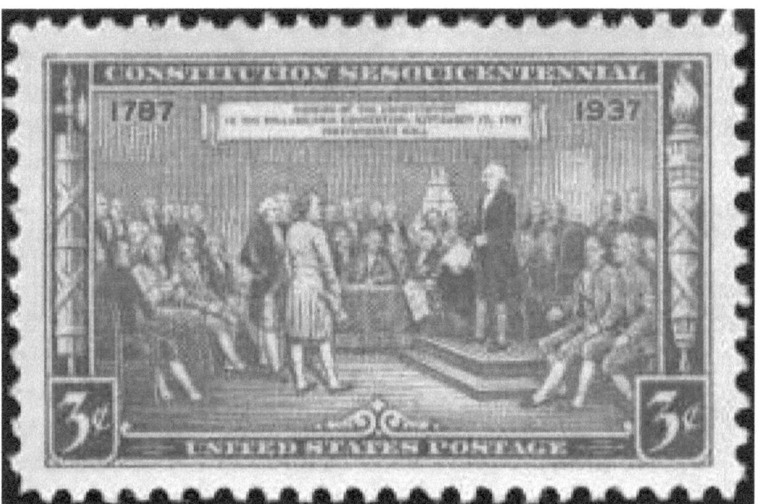

A stamp commemorating the signing of the Constitution The French Revolution

Maximilien Robespierre: "The secret to freedom is in educating people. But the secret to tyranny lies in keeping them ignorant."

   The reign of King Louis XVI and his wife Marie Antoinette was the low point in the history European monarchy. Her famous quote from that era, "Qu'ils mengent de la brioche", ("Let them eat cakes") is still a common one. While historians dispute the authenticity of this quote, it still serves to illustrate the distant cruelty of a close circle of hereditary monarchs.

   One could describe the French Revolution as a series of events and circumstances that culminated in the greatest uprising in human history. The Seven Years War and the American Revolution, which occurred two months prior to the French Revolution, left the French government in deep debt. In an attempt to balance the budget, various taxes were placed on an already poor population. The woes of France's masses were exacerbated by years of poor harvests and deregulation of grain production. The peasant population was pushed to the forefront by the conspicuous privilege enjoyed the nobility, the monarchy, and the senior clergy. The American Revolution, which was a popular movement that saw the overthrow of British control in 13 colonies, served to inspire French revolutionary leaders. It proved that it was possible to have such a bold dream as a modern republic. This combined with the Enlightenment ideals triggered the events that led to the overthrow of France's monarchy and the founding of the First Republic of France.

In 1791, the new revolutionized National Assembly created the first constitution of the Republic. All sovereignty was transferred to the Legislative Assembly. The members were elected through an indirect vote. Active citizen taxpayers made up about two-thirds (or three quarters) of all adult men. They were granted the right of vote for constituent members of an electoral College and for certain local officials. The 1791 constitution was only in force for a little over a year. It placed more emphasis on constitutionality than the rule of the kings. It was the result of many committees. In many ways, the constitution represented the futile efforts of a revolutionary dilletante coterie. The Third Estate, inspired and guided by the principles of government by people, attempted to draft the constitution. As a way to balance out the power of people and the potential influence of self-interest if the country was ruled only by representatives, the constitution granted the right of veto the king.

Although it was not an egalitarian constitution, it did provide a significant restriction on the executive power of the king. These events are called the Bourbon Restoration. They lasted only as long as the 1791 constitution. The Assemblee legislative was the place of authority, and it existed between October 1, 1791 and September 20, 1792. The king tried to exercise his right to veto against subjugation to the church by the government and refused to raise militias to defend the Revolutionary Government. He was then deposed in what became known as the "August 10, Insurrection." Maximilien Robespierre, who was elected by a National Convention to the post of First Deputy.

The first French assembly to be elected through universal male suffrage was the National Convention. It convened on September 20, 1792. France became a republic a few days later.

Although the First Republic was only able to survive for 12 years it was one of the most important 12 years in the nation's history. This chaotic, chaotic journey to popular sovereignty in France was filled with misadventures and crisis. August 19th 1792 saw a violent insurrection that was uncontrolled. The citizens of Paris stormed Tuileries Palace and killed 600 members of the Swiss Guards. They demanded the resignation of King Charles. In the countryside, anti-revolutionary movements were raging. Fearing the revolution, mobs stormed Paris' prisons in September 1792. They massacred many prisoners, including clergymen, nobles and political prisoners. This was the scene that became known as the September Massacres.

A National Convention was formed to draft a new constitution, and also to bring the king before a court after he had been stripped of all his political power. Louis, then a private citizen was brought before a court to be tried for high treason. This was one of the most controversial acts in the French Revolution. He was tried in December 1792 and convicted in January 1793. He was executed by guillotine.

The First Republic had one feature: the resolve of European monarchies to prevent it from being allowed to survive. This was the backdrop for the rise of Napoleon Bonaparte. The business of war was always a priority for Napoleon Bonaparte as he fought the War of the First Coalition. Paris was hit by food riots and widespread hunger in the following years. A Committee of Public Safety was formed in April 1793 to deal with unrest in the streets, various outbreaks of radical actions and Enrages and other crises that were affecting the capital. The Reign of Terror began when the main tool of suppression was the guillotine.

The violence and chaos of France's Revolution proved to nervous monarchies, who were watching from afar, that the peasants lacked the temperament and aptitude to govern. In 1793, a second constitution was drawn up. It was approved by the people in August. However, the Committee of Public Safety was continuing its work. Over 16,000 enemies were sent to the guillotine in the following year. Many thousands more died from mistreatment in various prisons.

Robespierre was executed on July 28, 1794. He was the brilliant ideologue of France's Revolution and the architect of the Reign of Terror. His power accumulation and relentless pursuit of anti-revolutionary support, which led to the horrendous spectacle of the Reign of Terror were his downfall.

One year after his execution and arrest, the National Convention adopted the Constitution of the Year III (August 22, 17,95), with its preamble including the following:

"declaration of the Rights and Duties of Man and of the Citizen of1795" Large numbers of political prisoners were freed and elections were held for a new legislative body. The Directory was established on November 3, 1795. For the next four-years, France was governed by the Directory, a committee of five members.

Napoleon, France's former enemy, invaded Ottoman Empire in 1799. He conquered modern Syria (then called the province of Damascus), and captured the cities of Gaza and Jaffa, Arish, and Haifa. Napoleon had to retreat after the plague ravaged his army and his supply lines from Egypt were too thin. He lost almost all his wounded when he fled from enemy forces. The majority of the wounded were tortured, and even beheaded.

Napoleon returned to Cairo with dispatches from France. The French had delayed sending them due to the fact that the Mediterranean was rife and full of Royal Navy vessels. The dispatches mentioned renewed hostilities between Austria and its allies and a series defeats in Italy that had effectively wiped out all Napoleon's hard-won gains on the Italian peninsula. Napoleon left his army under the command his subordinate General Kleber and embarked on one of his remaining ships. Napoleon set sail for France to rescue France from the new wave of enemies.

The situation was somewhat better by the time Napoleon arrived in France. The immediate threat of invasion was eliminated by a series of French victories along the country's borders. This included a decisive one against the Austrians, in the Alps, at the hands General Massena (one of Napoleon's pupils). The country was still rife in political tension. People viewed the newly formed Directory as ineffectual and supine. Their situation was made worse by years of war and an enemy naval blockade. France was open to change.

Napoleon was offered the chance to take part in that change by Emmanuel Sieyes, one of the Directors. He included Napoleon in his plan to put on a coup against Directory and seize power. Napoleon was not one to refuse a chance to advance. He took command of a detachment and led key members of the Directory from Paris to Chateau Saint Cloud, where he also escorted them away from their Paris seat. The Directory members realized that there was something suspicious going on and tried to protest. Napoleon ordered his men with bayonets to advance on them. Napoleon managed to persuade or convince most of the legislators to disperse and named himself, Sieyes, and Roger Ducos as temporary Consuls and effective rulers in France.

Emmanuel Sieyes always believed that Napoleon would be a subordinate figure in the governing the country. He was also grateful to have been involved in the plot. But Sieyes underestimated the man he was dealing. A little more than a month after the coup Napoleon wrote a constitution known as the Constitution of the Eighth Year of the Republic. This placed all legislative and executive power in the hands of the First Consultant and gave the two remaining subordinate positions. Napoleon, having already defeated foes on battlefield, displayed his political skills by outwitting Sieyes badly. Napoleon was elected First Consul and, thus, became the de facto monarch.

Napoleon, now in Paris, led an army to Italy in 1800. This campaign culminated in his victory over Austrian forces at Battle of Marengo. It was a rarely close-run engagement, whose outcome was determined by French reinforcements arriving in the eleventh hour. One need only see his plans for Marengo after the war to prove how crucial Napoleon thought this victory was. Napoleon gave his subordinates the task of building a pyramid to commemorate his victory. Streets would be named after his victories in Italy. The plans were canceled, but Napoleon did not lose sight of the significance of the victory. He would name the horse Marengo and ride Marengo in important battles such as Austerlitz or Waterloo.

Although the campaign ended all Austrian belligerence, a second campaign led by Napoleon's generals in Austria was required to end all resistance and impose The Treaty of Luneville upon the Austrians. This treaty confirmed all French territorial advances made before and after the Treaty of Campo Formio. Britain, without one of its strongest allies on the mainland, also decided to end hostilities and sign the Treaty of Amiens. However, this peace would be extremely short-lived.

Although Napoleon did not have the right to seek peace, he was forced to do so. Despite his victories France was still in debt and was vulnerable. Napoleon's position was also far from secure. Napoleon's political maneuverings had given him power but also made enemies from all sides, including Jacobins and Royalists. He foiled two plots against his life in 1800. Napoleon had also reinstituted slavery in France's colonies, but it proved to be ill-advised, as slaves in Saint Domingue, Haiti, and other countries rose up in revolt later in the year. A force sent to crush the rebellion was destroyed by yellow fever. Napoleon, conscious of the Clausewitzian maxim, "A general must not reinforce failure", was forced to surrender those possessions to rebels. In a desperate search for money, Napoleon sold large portions of France's North American holdings to the United States to help fill France's shrinking coffers. The Louisiana Purchase, which cost less than 3 cents an acre (or 40 cents in current currency), doubled America's size and still makes up over 20% of America today. Napoleon was seeking ways to finance the expansion of his empire and also had geopolitical reasons for the deal. Napoleon declared that the United States' power was forever assured by the accession to the territory he had acquired. He also gave his blessing.

England is a maritime competitor who will sooner or later humble her pride."

Napoleon did not want another long and costly war in 1803. He was allowed to revive France's finances but was forced to choose. In May 1803 Britain violated the Treaty of Amiens, declaring war on France. In fury at the turn of events, Napoleon began to build a massive army of around 200,000 men at Boulogne with the intention of crossing the Channel and invading England. Napoleon divided the army into seven corps with their own artillery units and a reserve cavalry that was then organized into divisions. This military organization was adopted by the rest of the world and is still used today, more than half a century after the American Civil War.

   Napoleon was acutely aware, despite this mobilization that his position in France wasn't stable. His spies stopped a Bourbon plot against Napoleon's murder and executed the Duke of Enghien. This was despite not having been involved in the plot. France's famed and erstwhile diplomat, Jean-Jacques Rousseau, advised him to make such a drastic move.

Talleyrand, the Foreign Minister, would be one of Napoleon's most influential advisers. Napoleon I was crowned Emperor of France at Notre Dame in December 1804, to make it more difficult for Bourbon to succeed to the throne. Napoleon was crowned King of Italy in Milan a few months later with another grand coronation. These actions allowed him to confer titles on his top generals and name them Marshals for the Empire to ensure their loyalty.

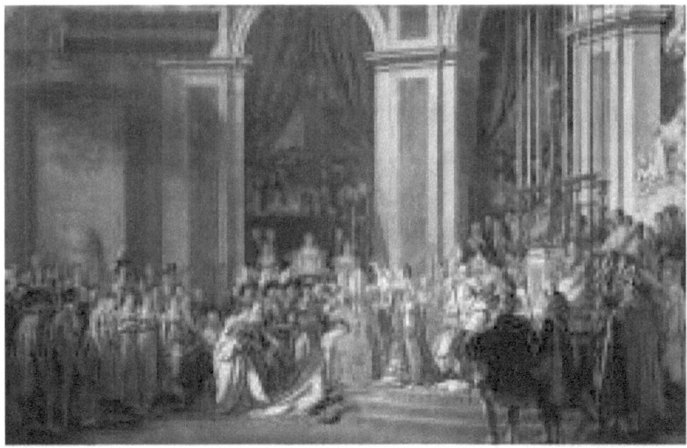

Coronation of Napoleon I and Empress Josephine by Jacques-Louis David, 1804

   Although the French Revolution sent shockwaves across Europe, despite Napoleon's creation an empire, it received mixed responses in Britain. The London Chronicle reported that the flame of liberty had erupted in every province of the great kingdom. It also stated that when a nation with an educated mind asserts its claim to the rights of men, it is not within the power of monarchs to deny them their right. France will be flooded with blood before they achieve their goal.

These words were prophetic, and they were repeated across the Atlantic. They also sounded a warning to anyone contemplating revolution at home. The French Revolution was generally celebrated in literary and artistic circles. It was also praised in many pamphlets and books that were published in England. Even as the guillotine weighed heavily on the necks and heads of the unfortunate and innocent, The Rights of Man by Thomas Paine in America was originally written as a history of the French Revolution and Mary Wollstonecraft's response to Edmund Burke's A Vindication of the Rights of Man.

Men published A Vindication of the Rights of Women (1790). Evidently, the events in France prompted a lot of reflection in Britain about how society was organized along class lines and by gender lines.

The French Revolution also sparked a reaction from the working class in England and the Kingdom. In 1792, the London Correspondence Society was founded to distribute information and propaganda and to encourage the working class to acknowledge the violence committed against their rights and unite them in the pursuit of regaining those rights.

With a deep sense for disquiet, the conservative establishment thought it over and created many opposing societies and organizations to claim wealth and class rights. The march towards universal liberty was somewhat accelerated by Britain, although the French Revolution inspired many to look at the state of British society. However, the transition towards reform would be relatively peaceful. Napoleon's proclamation as Emperor of France gave the ruling classes an opportunity to highlight the failures of the French Revolution's leaders. The eventual defeat at Waterloo of Napoleon would make Britain the greatest empire ever known.

The First Reform Act

"The elections clearly demonstrated to me that an Indian candidate has as good of a chance than any Englishman or has some advantages over one, because there is a genuine desire among English electors for India to receive any assistance in their power." – Dadabhai Naoroji

Unexpected things happened in the British General Election of 1892. The Liberal Party, which was the main opposition party, had a candidate from India for the inner-city London constituency Finsbury Central. To the delight of the Conservative political establishment, they won. Dadabhai Naoroji was only elected for one cycle. His role as an opposition backbencher wasn't particularly noteworthy, but the simple fact in 1892 that the British electorate was strong enough to allow an intellectual politician, from the outer reaches, to contest and win a parliamentary seat was a powerful message about the maturity and strength of the British metropolitan democracy system.

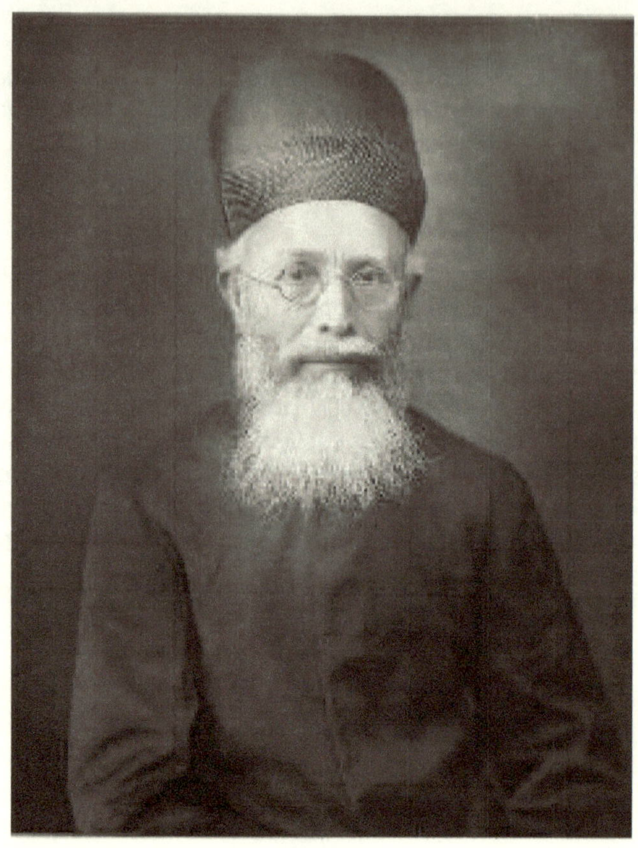

Naoroji

However, there was an irony to Dadabhai Naoroji's election. This was actually the point he was trying to make. Since the 1858 birth of the British Raj, the informal British imperial charter has stressed equality for all subjects of Her Majesty. The franchise, which was similar to the one in the United States, was very narrowly focused and often dependent on education and property. This had the effect of restricting access not only to large numbers of native inhabitants of the colonies, but also to the poor and uninformed working class of England. The territories of India and Ireland were governed as British colonies and were administered by the imperial governor at Whitehall. Indians were therefore denied the right to vote in their country. However, if they did qualify, they were allowed to vote in Britain.

Dadabhai Naoroji was certainly qualified as he was a Professor in the field of

Mathematics and Natural Philosophy at Elphinstone College, Bombay, as well as Gujarati at University College London. His decision to run for English public office was meant to emphasize this absurdity and to expose the British metropolitan public to the brightest and most talented Indians. He was not running as an Englishman of second class, but as an Indian of first class.

All of this being said, the culmination of an 60-year-old process of electoral reform in Britain was marked by the 1892 general election. The general, chaotic, and unregulated growth of the British electoral system led to many anomalies. This created a corrupt, cronyist system that existed for most of the past century under threat of reform. The "rotten and pockets boroughs" is a term used by reform advocates to refer to specific electoral constituencies in the United Kingdom that were under the control or a small group of electors. In whose pocket was the constituency, the "owner" of the borough could nominate any member of parliament he wanted. Sometimes, he was even able to auction off a constituency. For example, there were several constituencies along the coast that had been lost to the sea but that returned their members to Westminster. Two Members of Parliament were regularly represented Old Sarum, a hill uninhabited on the outskirts the English town Salisbury.

During the Industrial Revolution, the practical effects on the major British cities were transforming, and large numbers of tax-paying city dwellers were denied the right to vote. They were also growing frustrated at an archaic, tightly controlled system of politics. There were many examples of corruption and cronyism, which was generally agreed upon by the new intelligencesia. As with any system that is based on vested interests, reform was not desired by those who are most likely to benefit. Lord Arthur Wellesley, the Tory Prime Minister, was opposed to any discussion on parliamentary reform. However, he didn't speak for all members of his party. Many believed that the party loyal to the middle class would be able to exploit the wealth and influence of Britain's expanding middle class by responding to calls for at most a partial extension to the franchise.

There was growing support beyond the Tory Party for more radical parliamentary reform. After the initial shock of the French Revolution's violence had subsided, the message that remained in the minds working Britons was that Britain might also benefit from a radical overhaul to an outdated and degraded system was no longer relevant. In every area, from penal reform to abolishment, the Enlightenment tenets were being more widely accepted. Rapid industrialization created wealth. Education was followed by rapid growth of the printing presses. All of this led to a greater interest and understanding of the affairs of empire and state. The British were able to defeat Napoleon at Waterloo, establishing them as the leading European imperial power. As the British navy fleet was decommissioned, it turned its attention towards geographic exploration, Britain was redefining its place in the world. This was also when the first calls to include women in the franchise were made.

After King George IV's death, Parliament was disbanded and a general election called in 1830. The first time electoral reform was a major campaign rallying cry. Although the Tories were led at Waterloo by the Duke of Wellington (hero of Waterloo), divisions within Tory members over the issue of parliamentary reform grew. The party split so much that Earl Grey, an opposition Whig leader was able form a government. He was the one who led the nation to a second general elections in the next year with electoral reform dominating the campaign agenda. It was no surprise that the 1831 general election saw a strong victory for Whigs. This resulted in the final general election with an unreformed Parliament.

The year that followed was one of intense political maneuvering. Two failed reform bills were brought to the House before a third, the Representation and the People Act 1832, First Reform Act or the Great Reform Act, was passed. The First Reform Act made very little progress, but it opened the door to a continuing program of restructuring, which would lead to the Third Reform Act in 1884.

The First Reform Act, which was passed in England and Wales, drastically reduced the number of boroughs to 56. It also reduced the number members representing 30 more and created 67 new constituencies. The property qualification was expanded to include small landowners and tenant farmers, as well as minor tradesmen. This created a standard qualification of PS10 per monthly rental per householder. Although this was not affordable to the average farmer, peasant or urban worker, it did standardize and regulate the franchise, making the system more accessible to many more people. A second, less favorable addition to the Act's articles was the exclusion of women voting in Parliamentary elections. This specifically defined a voter as a "male person" under the terms in the Act.

It was evident to all that real change was possible. Although the empire's ruling class was content to accept that reform calls had been answered, the rising power of the working class in Britain was enough to convince Parliament that there was more to be done. The Chartist movement, which was highly influential, emerged in 1836 as the first genuine mass movement that was organized and led by the working class. It was born out of frustration over the failure to grant franchise rights to working class citizens by the 1832 Reform Act.

The London Working Men's Association drafted a People's Charter, listing six key demands. The first demand was universal male suffrage and the second was secret ballot. Equally important was the abolishment of property qualifications to run for Parliament, as well as various adjustments to terms and size. While petitions were presented and raised, Parliament refused to comply. In general, the era of mass mobilisation saw the traditional ruling classes of England under increasing siege. It was clear to all that reforms of the electoral system were needed by the time Chartist movements peaked in late 1850s. However, universal male suffrage was an obstacle that Parliament was unwilling to cross.

The Second Reform Act, which was passed in 1867, extended the franchise and nearly doubled the electorate of England and Wales to 1 million to 2,000,000 men. In 1884, the Third Reform Bill was introduced into Parliament.

William Gladstone was the Prime Minister. Parliamentary resistance to "one person one vote" was almost gone by that time. It was inevitable and common sense that the electorate was sophisticated enough to make it impossible to continue arguing against it. A strong urban middle class and empowered working class were hard to ignore. The rise of daily newspapers, expansion of the empire, as well as the expanding scope of education, created a society that was very interested in the affairs of the state at home and abroad. A uniform franchise was established across the country. There were a few technical adjustments made to constituencies and redistribution to seats. However, it reached a point where 60% of adult males living in England and Wales could vote.

This was the backdrop in which the Right Honourable Dadabhai Naoroji became the first British non-white member to Parliament. He won the election by the smallest margin, earning him the nickname of Narrow Majority (his name is Now-ohro-jai). In the same vein, the press seized on Mancherjee Bhownaggree (an Anglicized Hindu) as the next Indian to enter British politics. This conservative Tory viewed India's establishment as a co-worker. In the popular press, he was known as Bow-and -Agree.

However, the election of two Indians to the British Parliament in the early 20th century was seen by many as a victory of the Parliamentary Reform movement that had been incubating since 1832. However, the question of the imperial franchise remained at the core of dissonance between a liberal metropolitan voter willing to give an Indian chance and an overseas voter unwilling to allow it. As mentioned earlier, India had never been allowed to vote and, with the exception of minor reforms in 20th century, she has never been allowed to do so under British rule.

The rules were not as clear elsewhere. For example, in the Natal Colony where Mohandas Karmchand Gandhi, a young Indian politician, worked hard to gain free access to the franchise for his growing community, the British-dominated colonial legislature tried to stop him. India was governed by British colonial rule, but most British colonies that were settled at the end of 19th century had their own legislatures, premiers, and cabinets. This was true for the Natal Colony. The white community began to fear an Indian invasion because of the rapid growth of the Indian population, which was a result of free immigration and imported indentured labor.

The Colonial Secretary received a bill from the Natal Legislative Assembly in 1894. It was called the Natal Franchise Bill. This bill specifically sought to exempt Indians from the colony's vote. The Colonial Secretary was unable to approve the bill and sent it back to Durban. He recommended that any reference to race be removed from the document before Her Majesty could be approved. After pondering this problem for some time, the Natal committee drafted the bill. It then returned it to Whitehall with a minor modification to the language. The draft stated that any resident of Natal without access to their home colony's vote would be allowed to vote in Natal. The bill was passed and signed into law. Indians are now denied the right to vote in the Natal Colony, as it did not make any mention of race.

The situation was quite different in the Cape colony. The Cape, a self-governing colony also had a large population of English-speaking and Dutch-speaking liberals. Their colonial constitution provided for full access to the franchise to all men, regardless of race, color or creed. It was granted this right based on the same essential property as Britain and the same education qualifications. At the time, the Cape's "colourblind" constitution was considered the highest example of a liberal colonial constitution. It was the only one like it anywhere. It survived, and was diligently protected until white Afrikaner nationalism began to gradually erode its fundamental elements. This was probably the most striking example of British imperial impartiality at its best.

The British reform movement had largely ended, but a small percentage of British males were still denied the right to vote due to their education and property qualifications. Just before the end World War I, the 1918 Representation Act of the People was passed. It finally eliminated all qualifications for males older than 21 years. They only needed proof of identity to vote. Women were also granted the right to vote for the first time, but they had to meet stringent requirements.

15 years ago, Lord Glasgow, Governor of New Zealand signed a new Electoral Act. This liberalized local electoral laws. New Zealand is the only modern democratic country (albeit still a colonial) that grants women the right of vote. This was a victory for the strong local suffragist movement, led by Kate Sheppard, a feminist political campaigner. New Zealand was inspired by the larger suffrage movements in all major democracies around the globe and led the charge in the next major battle for universal adult voting rights.

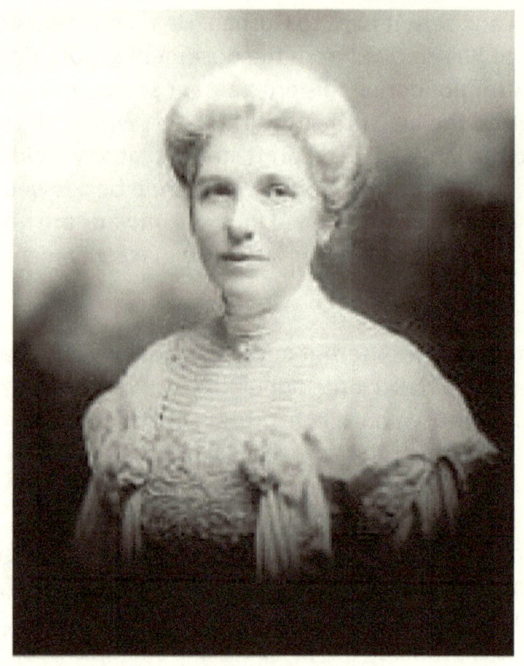

Sheppard

Suffrage Movements

You must make women count equally as men. Women must be given political power to ensure that the law of the land reflects their moral standards. It's the only way." Emmeline Pankhurst

The First Reform Act of 1832 began a process that would end in

February 1918, with full enfranchisement for all male population

Britain. Women would not be tortured in any of these cases.

While the Parliamentary debates brought about all this, a few politically active women remained vigilant and started to plan their campaign to win the vote.

It was not just a very few men who thought of extending the franchise to women, but it also seemed to be very few women. The majority of women did not support the leaders of the early suffrage movements in Britain and America. As the struggle to expand the franchise's access began, however, more women began to become active behind the scenes and movements for female suffrage began to gain momentum.

However, women are not politically inactive because there were no major suffrage movements before. Women on both sides of the Atlantic were more likely to be the driving force behind the grassroots abolition movement. Feminism as an ideology evolved from a growing awareness of human rights and social reform. Women were involved in issues such as war and penal reform, and could be found as far as South Africa and the Crimea assisting with the terrible collateral effects of war. Their struggle for the franchise was the most important moment in democratic history and was the final step towards universal adult suffrage.

Victorian Era saw women idolized in an era of exaggerated knighthood, when the man's role was to worship and defend and the woman's role was to worship and be protected. Anecdotal accounts of women hiding their intelligence to preserve their status in life and not appear to be a threat for men are common in this era. This convention was not challenged by many women, and those who did were most likely doing so at their own peril.

In the early days of the franchise, the reasons women were denied voting rights were less a matter for law than convention. Women were considered essentially wards of their husbands or fathers. If the question was ever posed, it would likely be that the system shouldn't bother to duplicate the vote of a man by allowing his spouse to vote. A married couple was considered two halves of one whole. Victorian women were also considered impractical and weak-minded, possibly excepting Queen Victoria. This theory was clearly disproven by the fact that so few people were educated beyond a basic level.

In the latter part of the 19th century, a lot of women began to protest this issue. England's factories were full of working women, who paid rates and taxes and were subject to the laws of England. They no longer considered themselves as economic extensions of their husbands. Soon, informal organizations emerged and the name "suffragist" was given to the movement.

There were many suffragist groups in the United Kingdom with the common goal of securing the right to vote through peaceful and constitutional means. The National Union of Women's Suffrage Societies (or the NUWSS) was the first national organization. It was founded in 1897 by Millicent Fawcett (52) and is the first British feminist activist to have a national profile. Millicent Fawcett, a prolific lobbyist, speaker, and campaigner, was married to Henry Fawcett (a Liberal MP who was blind) and was one of few Victorian politicians who relied on a practical, public partnership with his wife.

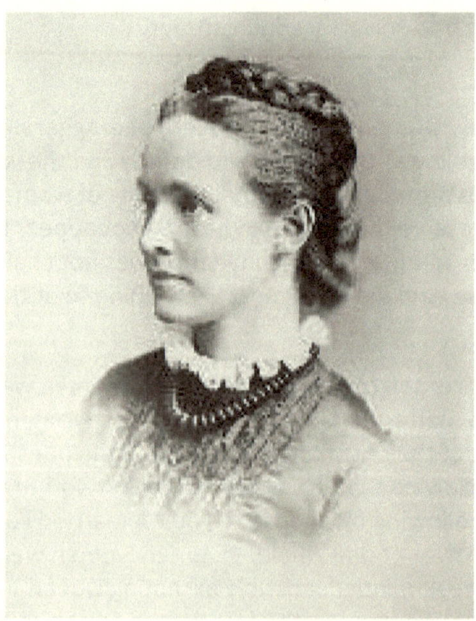

Millicent Fawcett

Millicent Fawcett, in her own right was a passionate campaigner but also a skilled and guileful tactician. She was a Victorian-style politician, but she managed to steer the NUWSS towards national prominence. She was well-connected in the Parliamentary fraternity of the time. She and many deputies and campaigners worked hard for the promotion of their campaign to gain sympathy from MPs and to bring to the floor numerous debates about women's suffrage.

Since then, the organization has been criticised for focusing its efforts on the elite progressive middle-class women and lobbying Parliament at great cost to efforts to build mass support among rural and working-class females. At the turn of this century, 58% of male citizens could vote. There was a feeling that men with lower socioeconomic status would not be allowed to vote and it was futile to campaign for their rights.

Each of the Reform Acts were being steered through Parliament. A petition was submitted to the House of Commons asking for the inclusion of the question of women's votes in the discussion. For example, in 1866, the Women's Suffrage Committee, headed by Barbara Bodichon, was formed by a veteran campaigner. It was established by a petition that John Stuart Mill, Liberal philosopher and political economist, presented to Parliament. The petition included 1,500 names. Although a list of 1,500 names is very small, it's important to remember that Barbara Bodichon was part of a close circle of upper middle-class and noble women living in the capital of the country. 1,500 was a solid base of support.

In the meantime, the Suffrage Movement was gaining a militant tone. This coincided with Emmeline Pankhurst, a Mancunian woman aged 40, becoming more prominent. She was born July 15, 1858, one day after the anniversary for the storming at the Bastille. She remarked in 1908 that she believed that her birth on July 15, 1858 had a certain influence on her life. [7]

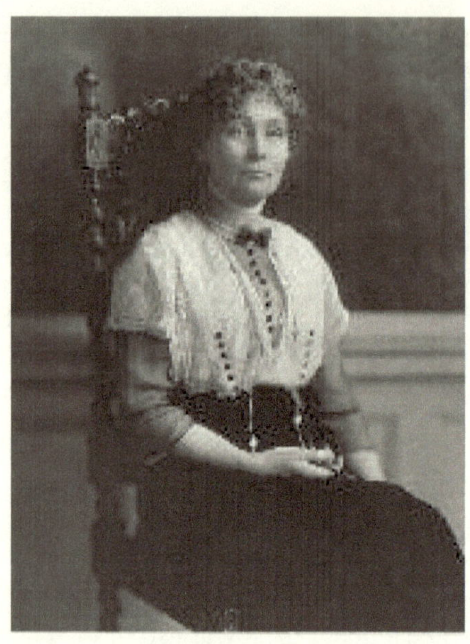

Pankhurst

On October 10, 1903 at 62 Nelson Street in Manchester, the home and office of

Emmeline Pankhurst was the founder of the militant Women's Social and Political Union. Its founder members were Emily Pankhurst and her two daughters, Sylvia and Christabel Pankhurst. Its motto was "deeds and not words", which was a clear expression of frustration. The WSPU was organized quickly, attracted a large membership, and campaigned with a message that was unrestrained activism. Although peaceful and constitutional means had achieved some public awareness, the WSPU members set out to make the message more powerful.

Initial disruptions and civil disobedience were the basis for a campaign of positive actions. This earned the group the derogatory name of the "suffragettes", which was quickly adopted by the movement. In October 1908, an organized attempt to invade Parliament was launched. Despite the presence of around 60,000 people in Parliament Square, near the palace's main entrance, a police line prevented the invasion. After being struck by King George V's horse, Anmer, during the Epsom Derby in June 1913, Emily Davison, a suffragette, died. She had been trying to attach a badge about women's rights to the horse's neck, but the common version says she was trying. Emily Davison's death is perhaps the most famous image of the suffragette movement.

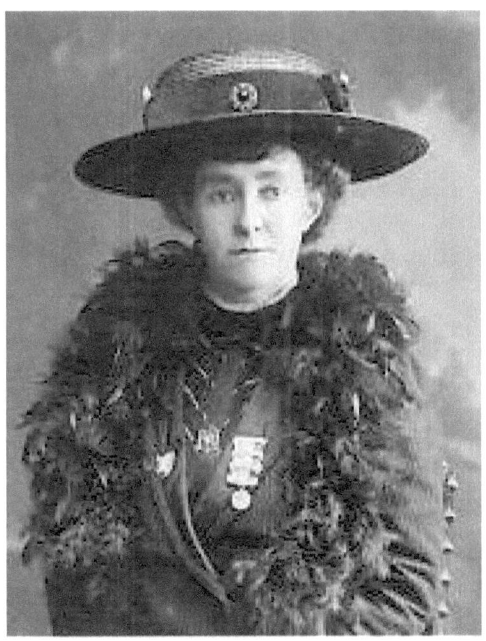

Davison

The message was clear: women wanted the vote. But the political establishment resisted. Violent protests, hunger strikes, law-breaking, and attacks on property followed. All of these helped to spread the message and attract more support. The establishment began to realize that there was a mass movement. Although the outbreak of World War I temporarily halted suffragette activities, it had a much greater impact on the generation of sympathy for the feminist movement and the suffrage movement. This was because women were immediately able to join the workforce to do "men's work", as the majority of the nation's men marched off to war. By 1918, the guns had stopped, there was much greater acceptance within the political establishment of the equality and contributions made by women.

The 1918 Representation of People Act opened up the doors slightly to women. Qualified franchise was available to anyone over 30. Although 8.5

million women were eligible for this qualification, it still represented a fundamental inequality. This is especially because the same act eliminated all educational and property qualifications for men. Protests continued, and many were more violent, but the signs were on the wall in all respects. A decade later, in 1928 the Equal Franchise Act was passed and universal adult suffrage became a reality in the United Kingdom.

American Suffragettes

On August 18, 1920, across the Atlantic, in the United States, the

The Nineteenth Amendment to the Constitution of the United States was approved, giving women the right of vote. This was the culmination a long-running process that was linked to various civil rights movements going back to the 19th century.

In 1848, Seneca Falls, New York hosted a benchmark conference that agreed that women were independent individuals and deserving of their political identities. Based on the American Declaration of Independence, a Declaration of Sentiments was created. It stated that "When human events make it necessary for one part of the family of men to assume among people of the earth an office that is different from the one they had previously held, but which the laws of God and nature allow them to hold, a decent respect for the opinions of humanity requires that they declare the reasons that have led them to this position." These truths are self-evident. All men and women are equal.

The Declaration of Sentiments concludes with these words: "Now in view of this whole disfranchisement of one half the people of this nation, their social, religious degradation--in light of the unjust laws mentioned, and because women feel themselves aggrieved and oppressed and fraudulently deprived of most sacred rights, insist that they have immediate access to all rights and privileges that belong to them as citizens of United States. "

In Worcester, Massachusetts, was held the first ever National Women's Rights Convention. Horace Greeley, a famous newspaper columnist, gave a fascinating account of Lucy Stone's speech. Stone's quote was just what

Susan B. Anthony needed to get her to the suffrage cause. We desire that she achieves the full development of her nature, and her womanhood. It may not be written on her tombstone that she is a'relict'.

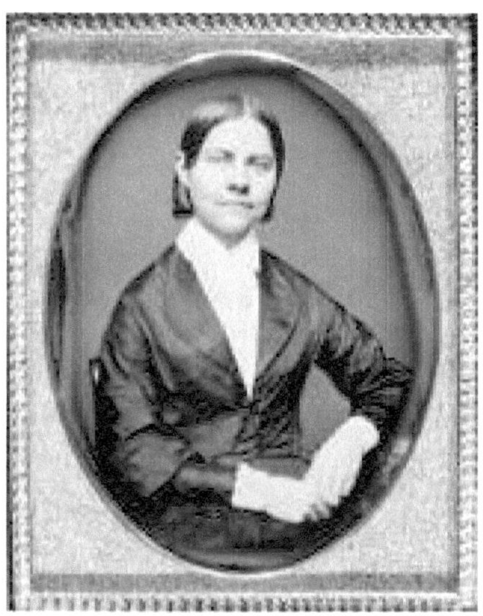

Lucy Stone

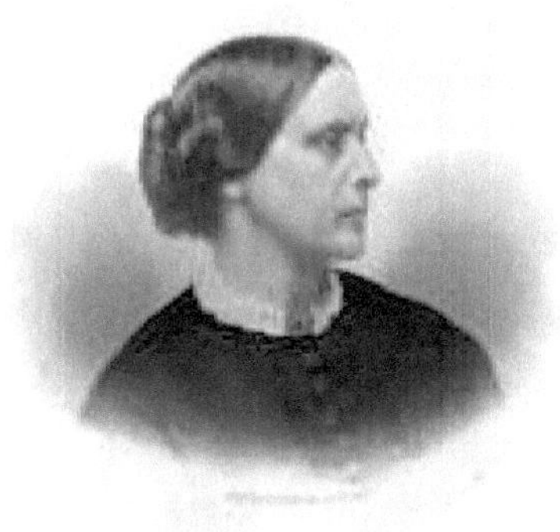

Susan B. Anthony

The abolition movement was inextricably linked to the movement to ensure women's right to vote. Many Americans have opposed slavery since colonial times. For many abolitionists slavery was the most important moral issue of the time. Their opposition was deeply rooted in their religious beliefs. Quakers were a key part of the colonial abolitionist movement. Other prominent opponents to slavery relied on natural law and Enlightenment ideals. Many Quakers and other abolitionists centered their efforts during colonial times on abolishing slavery in the northern colonies, and persuading slaveholders to release their slaves. Both of these efforts were successful and slaves were liberated in both the northern colonies and border slave states such as Delaware. The fact that tobacco cultivation was declining in the Mid-Atlantic slave state of Delaware, Maryland, and Virginia helped slaveholders convince them to release their slaves.

Anthony and Elizabeth Cady Stanton went on a speaking tour in New York to promote the message "No Union with Slaveholders" when the Civil War broke out. No Compromise." Anthony challenged her audience in one of her most stirring speeches:

"Let's, my friends, for this passing hour, make slave's cases our own. Let us not only believe in ourselves but also in our family members who have been despoiled of their inalienable rights of life, liberty, and the pursuit and pursuit of happiness. We must feel that our backs are being whipped by the slave driver. It is our flesh that is torn and lacerated. It is our blood that is poured out.

Let us remember that these are our children. They are driven through the burning suns and rains to join the "coffle Gang" and sold to the highest bidder. Then, they get rehabilitated and rebuilt on the rice, sugar, and cotton plantations in the remote south.

"Could you, my friends but make the slave's situation our own-- could you but feel for him, as bound with him (Heb13:3)? Could we not make him our neighbor and 'love him like ourselves' (Mt 22.39) and do unto him what we would do unto others (Lk 6.31)? How easy would it be to convert us all to Abolitionism.

"If a magic power could instantly change the color of our skins and make the fate of the slave ours, then there would be no need for argument, persuasion, rhetoric, or eloquence. With heart, soul, tone, and action, we would all respond to the truthfulness and justice of the glorious doctrine 'immediate, unconditional emancipation' as the right and duty of the slaves. Were we the victims of the most vile oppression that the sun has ever shine upon? No appeal to the Bible, Constitution, no respect for peace and harmony within our religious or political affiliations, no blind reverence in "Union" in either church or state could stop our actions, quieten our consciences, or silence our voices.

"All, all of them will sink into utter insignificance. Freedom, God's unfailing boon to mankind, is greater than all of them. "Liberty, or death" is our new watchword.

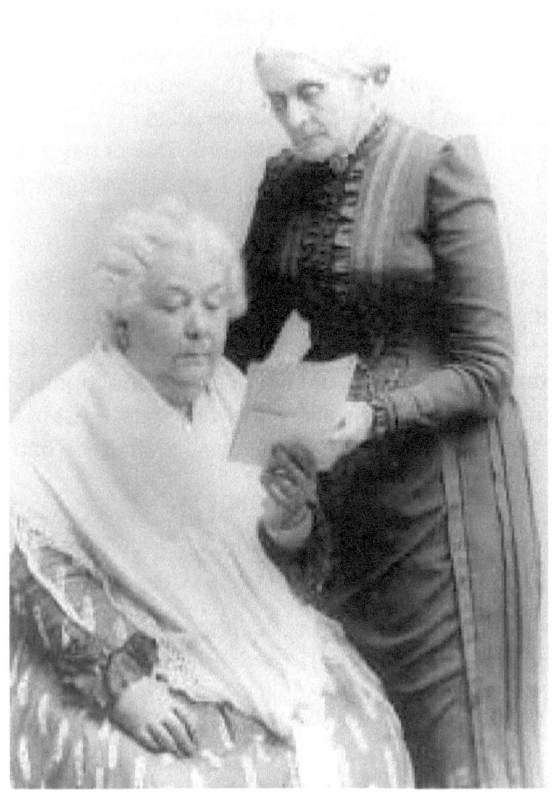

Elizabeth Cady Stanton and Susan B. Anthony

Stanton and Anthony devoted their efforts to the Union's defeat of the South during the Civil War years. They formed the Women's Loyal League with other suffragists to support President Lincoln's plans. In 1863, the women co-authored An Appeal to the Women of the Republic. This appeal urged women to stand firm for the Union and support it in all ways. They supported the Thirteenth Amendment's passage, which would legalize slavery as an official act of war. A year later, the Fourteenth Amendment was ratified. It further defined citizenship rights and guaranteed equal protection. The Fifteenth Amendment made it illegal to deny a man the right to vote on the basis of race, color, or a previous condition of servitude.

Anthony and Stanton saw a chance to extend the voting rights to women with the Fifteenth Amendment, which gave former slaves the right of vote. They formed the American Equal Rights Association (AERA), on May 10, 1866 at the Eleventh National Woman's Rights Convention. The association's sole purpose was to promote legislation that would allow both African Americans and women to vote. Anthony would exhort: "I beg of you to speak of Woman like you do about the Negro. Talk of her as a human being and citizen of the United States. In whose hands lies this Nation's destiny."

Stanton and Anthony insisted that women have the right to vote with black men. They eventually started lobbying against Civil War Amendments in the current form. This only extended the voting rights to black men. Stanton and Anthony were shocked when fellow abolitionists with whom they had fought for the end of slavery showed no interest in helping women get the same rights as the men, even the black men, they had liberated.

Anthony was more pragmatic than Stanton, who was more zealous and called into question the abilities of others to vote:

"If the party in ascendency makes its demand to 'negro' suffrage in good faith, on grounds of natural right, and because it is in the best interests of the State that the republican idea should be vindicated, the women of this nation cannot be ignored on any principle of justice or safety.

"Considering the fact that the Freedmen from the South and the millions upon millions of foreigners who now crowd our Western shores are not property, education or civilization, it is in the best interest of the nation that we outweigh this incoming poverty, ignorance, degradation with the wealth, education and refinement that the women of republic have,

Frederick Douglas, an abolitionist, disagreed with Stanton. He maintained that white women had some political influence because they could influence the votes of men in their lives. This was unlike any African American. He was joined by Julia Ward Howe and Lucy Stone, female abolitionists. The fight for the vote ended the long-standing friendship between Frederick Douglass and the women. Alma Lutz, historian, says that the following incident took place at AERA Convention 1869:

Frederick Douglass, in his resolution endorsing Fifteenth Amendment, quoted Julia Ward Howe, who said, "I am willing the Negro shall receive the ballot before I," and then added, "I can't see how anyone could pretend that there is the exact same urgency in giving ballot to the women as the Negro."

"Quickly, Susan was up and on her feet challenging him. As the champion of women debated the question ...,, their friendship and warmth over the years sometimes shone through the harsh words they exchanged.

Susan stated that "The antislavery school used to say that women should stand aside." She also said that they should wait until the male Negroes become voters. We say that if you don't want to give justice to all people, then give it to the intelligentst first.

"Here she received applause. She continued: 'If intelligence and justice and morality are to go in the government then let the question about women be raised first .... Mr. Douglass discusses the wrongs committed by the Negro and how he is being hunted ...,. But with all the outrages and wrongs he currently suffers, he wouldn't exchange his sex for Elizabeth Cady.

Stanton.'

Frederick Douglass shouted, "I want to know, Frederick Douglass," "If granting you the right to vote will change the nature our sexes?"

Susan replied, "It will alter the pecuniary situation of woman," before the laughter subsided. "She won't be forced to accept only those jobs that man chooses for herself."

Stanton and Anthony created the National Woman Suffrage Association in 1869. This creed stated that "Universal Manhood Sufrage" imposes on women of the nation an absolute and cruel despotism rather than monarchy. In this, women find a political master in their husbands, fathers, brothers, and sons. Stanton was made the first president at Anthony's insistence and requested that the first national Woman Suffrage Convention be held in Washington D.C. in the year 1869. The meeting saw a split between the NWSA and the American Woman Suffrage Association. This would allow women to vote in federal elections. The first victory was Wyoming in the same year.

Stanton and Anthony started The Revolution, a feminist newspaper to help them get their message across. George Francis Train, a wealthy philanthropist, provided $600 to help them start the paper. Anthony convinced Andrew Johnson, the President of the United States of America, to purchase a subscription at $2.00 per annum.

Its masthead stated all they thought: "The true republic---Men have their rights, and nothing else; women have their rights, but nothing less." Stanton was the Editor-in-Chief and Anthony was the publisher. The Revolution advocated for eight hours of work and the purchase of goods made in America, rather than imported from abroad. They also supported immigration to repopulate and settle the West.

The Revolution was also the first publication to tackle the controversial issue of abortion head-on. It is not surprising that those who still argue the issue use Anthony's writings to support their case. The article, which was only signed "A" at the end of The Revolution, stated that "Guilty?" Yes. The woman who does the deed is guilty of a terrible crime, regardless of her motive. It will weigh on her conscience and her soul in the end. But, oh, thrice guilty was he who drove her towards the crime !... We want prevention, not punishment. It is done by those who are unable to stop the evil from being done. Although historians debate whether Anthony actually wrote it, she often signed her articles.

"S.B.A."

After Train's support ran out, it was difficult for the women to maintain their high moral standards. Stanton, Anthony insisted that the best printing be done and they hired women whenever possible to pay them a higher wage than usual. They refused to accept advertising for any immoral products, even those made by quack doctors. The paper soon fell behind due to insufficient advertising revenue.

Anthony also founded the Working Women's Association, which supports women in publishing and garment manufacturing. Anthony was able to welcome both African American and white women into his organizations in a revolutionary move. They campaigned for shorter work hours, a lower minimum age, and equal pay for all women.

Anthony initially believed that the Women's Movement was a natural alliance with the Labor Movement. Stanton and Anthony were soon to discover the truth when they were sent as delegate(s) to the National Labor Union Convention 1868. They discovered that the middle classes saw women's rights as a more important issue than they should be. Anthony made another mistake when she suggested that women could reach financial independence by getting into the printing business. She was unaware that the male printers were on strike, and they voted to expel Anthony from the meeting.

Stanton was elected the first woman to be elected to the United States Congress from New York in the same year. Stanton supported the rights for women to divorce their abusive husbands and to have custody of the children if they do so. She also supported the right for women to work in the same jobs as men. Stanton's views on abortion remain controversial, but they are clear. Stanton wrote to Julia Ward Howe, 1873, "When women are treated like property, it is degrading for women that we treat our children as property to disposed of as you see fit."

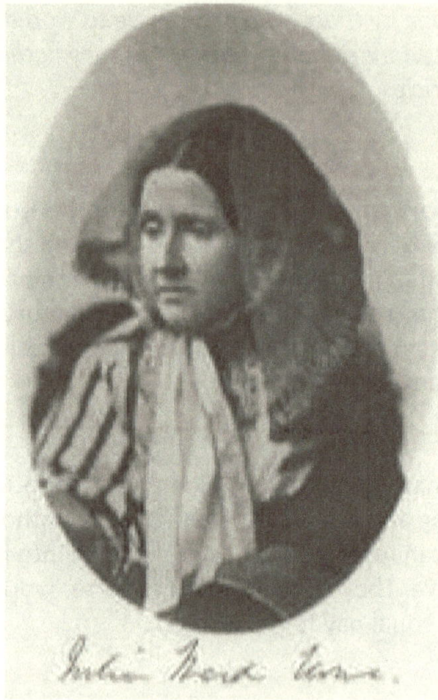

Julia Ward Howe

Stanton received an important letter from Anthony on November 5, 1872. Anthony had grown tired of just speaking and writing for Women's Suffrage. She decided, with her three sisters, to vote in the presidential election of November 5, 1872, regardless of whether it was legal.

Anthony was able to handle more speaking engagements in the time between her arrest and her trial. Anthony traveled to each county in which she was to be tried, and she spoke on the same topic: "Is It a Crime for a Citizen to Vote in the United States?" She quoted documents, laws, and Founding Fathers to prove that women should be allowed to vote.

Stanton, Anthony and Matilda Gage agreed in 1881 that it was time for future generations to record the efforts they made to ensure freedoms for their children and grandchildren. They began work on the History of Woman Suffrage together with Matilda Gage. Six volumes of the history were published by their successors in 1922.

Though Stanton never held political office in the United States, she did gain increasing notoriety in other parts of the world during her later years. With her daughter, Harriot Blatch, by her side, they spoke to both large and small groups of women on the progress of suffrage in America. They also helped organize the International Council of Women, which met for the first time in Washington, D.C. in 1888.

When she joined Anthony, Stone and Isabella Beecher Hooker in addressing the U. S. House Judiciary Committee in early 1892, even Stanton had to admit that they had "come a long way." The women were well received by the committee members and treated with the utmost respect. Part of the reason for this change was that, by this time, several states had already granted women the right to vote, so the handwriting seemed to be on the wall. In her testimony, Stanton made the following impassioned plea: "The isolation of every human soul and the necessity of self-dependence must give each individual the right to choose his own surroundings. The strongest reason for giving woman all the opportunities for higher education, for the full development of her faculties, her forces of mind and body; for giving her the most enlarged freedom of thought and action; a complete emancipation from all forms of bondage, of custom, dependence, superstition; from all the crippling influences of fear—is the solitude and personal responsibility of her own individual life. The strongest reason why we ask for woman a voice in the government under which she lives; in the religion she is asked to believe; equality in social life, where she is the chief factor; a place in the trades and professions, where she may earn her bread, is because of her birthright to self-sovereignty; because, as an individual, she must rely on herself..."

Elizabeth Cady Stanton died quietly in her home in New York City on October 26, 1902, nearly two decades before her dream of women having the right to vote in the United States. Ironically, Stanton's outspoken views and methods resulted in her legacy being tampered down. Her views about religion and her focus on other issues led women suffragists to make Susan B. Anthony the historical face of their movement. In 1923, when the 75th anniversary of the Seneca Falls Convention was commemorated, it fell upon Elizabeth's daughter Harriot to mention the role her mother had played. Despite the fact Stanton had been the instrumental leader at Seneca Falls, and the one who drafted the Declaration of Sentiments, posterity remembered Anthony as the founder of the women's rights movement. It was only in the last 35 years that history has properly revised itself to acknowledge the central role Stanton played in the movement.

Meanwhile, at the advanced age of 84, Anthony made her second trip to Europe in 1895, this time to Berlin, Germany, where she presided over the International Council of Women. While there she also served as the honorary president of the International Woman Suffrage Alliance. When she returned to the United States, she went to Washington, D.C., where she met with President Theodore Roosevelt and asked him to submit a suffrage amendment to Congress. Though he did not make any promises, he was kind and genial to his honored guest.

Anthony returned to Washington the following year to attend Congressional hearings on suffrage and to attend a celebration in honor of her 86th birthday on February 18th. She ended her final speech by assuring her audience "I am here for a little time only and then my place will be filled. But the fight must not cease. You must see that it does not stop. Failure is impossible." She received a 10-minute-long standing ovation.

Within a month, Anthony died at her home on Madison Street in Rochester on March 13. As she had correctly predicted, she did not live to see women get the right to vote. But it did occur within a generation. In 1920, 14 years after her death, the United States passed the Nineteenth Amendment to the Constitution. Known as the Susan B. Anthony Amendment, it gave every woman over 21 the right to vote in any federal election.

The End of the Empires

"To be free is not merely to cast off one's chains, but to live in a way that respects and enhances the freedom of others." – Nelson Mandela

The ratification of the Fifteenth Amendment was certainly a moment to celebrate, but in many respects it was only the beginning of a long road that led to the Civil Rights Movement in the 1960s. Even that represents less than the full story, because there were other places where black people were fighting for the right to vote. In the late 19th century, the first stirrings of political ambitions in Africa were setting the stage for the revolutions that would define the African liberation movement.

There were radically different approaches to the question of the non-white franchise in South Africa on the part of the two British colonies of that region. South Africa, however, comprised four white-ruled territories, two Boer republics – where no question of non-white representation was entertained at all – and two British colonies, where the franchise laws of Britain theoretically prevailed. The same was true in New Zealand and Australia, where both Māori and Aboriginal people theoretically enjoyed the right to vote and in many cases did, notwithstanding some localized manipulation of the rules. The signature difference between the British colonies of the South Pacific and those of Africa was simply that the indigenous populations of the former colonies never existed in any numbers to threaten the white man at the ballot box, while in Africa they certainly did.

Prior to the mid-19th century, there was very little interest expressed by the major European powers in the colonization of Africa. British and Dutch settlement of the southern African region had more to do with strategic naval interests than with any long-term occupation. The discovery of gold and diamonds in massive quantities towards the end of the 1870s changed this, and almost overnight South Africa became the center of British capital investment. The Boer, Dutch-speaking element of the white population was considerably older, more oriented towards the land, and a great deal more prejudicial with regards to entertaining any hint of black political ambition.

At the time, the indigenous population of sub-Saharan Africa was not in any position to challenge or threaten the gradual advance of European interest on the continent. Without written language or any of the fundamentals of invention or technology, they simply yielded to the greater power of Europe, and by the turn of the 20th century, the African continent was occupied in almost absolute totality. West and Equatorial Africa was dominated by the French, with a handful of notable exceptions, such as British Nigeria, while Britain controlled southern Africa, sharing East Africa with the Germans.
Belgium claimed the vast territory of the Congo while the two major Portuguese overseas dominions were Mozambique and Angola, with a handful of minor islands and colonies distributed elsewhere.

Each of these colonizing powers took a different view of their disenfranchised majority. The French adopted a system of grooming the black elites of their colonies and creating a separate class of assimilated blacks given full citizenship rights and welcomed into the representative bodies of the metropolitan capital. From as early as 1914, black representatives of the *communes* of Senegal were seated in the French Chamber of Deputies, while others were encouraged to enter French society and make use of the opportunities for education and cultural assimilation in France. These opportunities were not only available to the African *élites,* but also those from the Caribbean and other French colonies scattered around the world. The idea was to create two distinct classes, the *originaires,* or the residents of the communes, and the *indigène*, comprising everyone else excluded from the rights of assimilation. Only the former could vote.

The British, on the other hand, lumped everyone together as a subject of His or Her Majesty, leaving it to the colonial authorities to work out the messy details of who could vote and who could not. The imperial structure, however, only permitted the franchise in self-governing colonies, which were the white-settled colonies. The others were typically crown colonies or protectorates, run directly by the Secretary of State for the Colonies with no local system of the franchise at all. Likewise, the German and Belgian colonies offered no scope for black involvement other than at the lowest levels of administration, while Portugal, which regarded its colonies as overseas provinces, adopted a similar system to the French of cultivated elites.

The net result of it all was almost absolute disenfranchisement of a vast majority of blacks. In some cases, most notably the French, a phased and selective introduction to parliamentary politics was attempted, but this certainly held little advantage for the majority of the people.

The flagship of the British Empire was India, and it too contained the largest population. It is also true that India was home to perhaps the most sophisticated non-white population in the entire British Empire. Some of mankind's earliest traditions of representative rule originated in India, and if the people in territories like Australia and New Zealand were "civilized" enough that the British believed they deserved self-government, then Indians certainly deserved the same treatment.

At the same time, it was understood in Whitehall that the first bill to be debated in a homegrown legislature in India would be one authorizing the removal of the territory from the British Empire. The Indian Home Rule movement was led by certain seminal figures, such as the aforementioned Dadabhai Naoroji and Mohandas Gandhi, alongside a wide Congress membership of educated and professional men. By the turn of the 20th century, those Britons with any sort of sense of clarity realized that the loss of India to the empire was simply a matter of time, but as war clouds gathered over Europe, it was understood by both sides that it was in their common interest to weather that particular storm before attempting a separation. The nationalist movement eventually had to concede that in exchange for Indian commitment to imperial defense, Indian independence would be on the table the moment the fighting stopped.

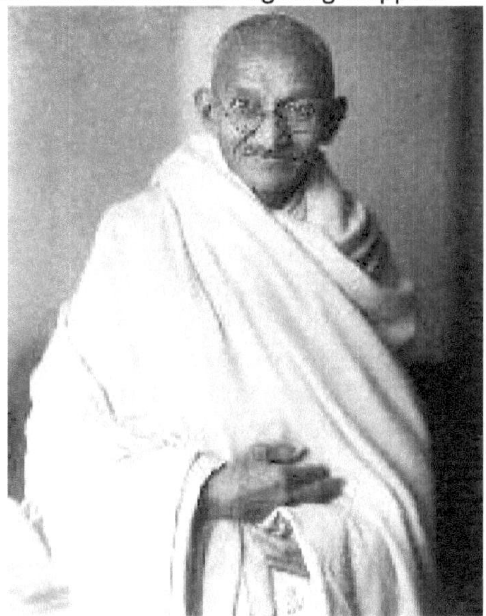

Gandhi

As it turned out, things did not quite work out that way, and a combination

of British imperial foot-dragging and Indian sectarian divisions tended to draw India's independence out until within two decades the clouds of another war hung heavy over Europe. This time the Indians faced the threat of a Japanese invasion and were less keen to throw out the British, even as the question of independence was one that really could no longer be ignored.

The difficulty lay with the fundamental incompatibility of Hindus and Muslims in India. By 1945, the writing was clearly on the wall for both the French and British, and both empires were keen to divest imperial responsibility in exchange for some sort of commonwealth of nations. India would be the first, and the British no longer had any appetite to endlessly wrangle over the details. The likes of Gandhi pleaded for Indian unity, and in the end that cost him his life. Eventually it was accepted as inevitable that India would be partitioned, creating the two states of India and Pakistan. The separation of the two territories was nothing if not traumatic, resulting in violence on an unprecedented scale. The handover of power in India took place on August 15, 1947, and as the British administration boarded ships and made their way home, India erupted into a firestorm. An untold number of people were killed, and India and Pakistan remain adversaries over 70 years later.

The net result was the creation of the biggest democracy in the world to date, but there were enormous consequences that few paid much attention to at the time. World War II had been fought by an Allied army comprised of troops from almost every corner of the British Empire. African troops fought in diverse theatres, but where they were most concentrated and most successful was in the Southeast Asian theatre. As an Axis defeat in Europe became an inevitability, Allied attention was focused on Burma, where the Japanese had been knocking on the door of India since their occupation. The Japanese were also on the run by then, and all that was really required was a concentrated push to send them on their way. The bulk of the army that dealt with this job was Indian, but a great many Africans were also involved. During initial deployment, furlough, and retraining, African battalions were almost all billeted at one time or another in India, and there they began to absorb the concepts of liberation that were so alive in Indian society at the time. This, in combination with the ideology underlining the defeat of fascism, caused many of these young men to return to their home colonies in Africa deeply inspired by what they had seen and heard, only to be brutally disabused when it became clear that none of those lofty ideals were intended to apply to them.

At precisely the same time, the first generation of highly educated black youth was filtering back from local and overseas universities, bringing with them the first crop of doctorates and master's degrees, most often earned by begging and borrowing, and with a minimum of assistance from the colonial establishment. This was true across the board, and not just in British colonies. One can time the moment that the African liberation movement began to when these two groups met. The returning soldiers provided the manpower, and the young, radical intellectuals the leadership. Very quickly the first indigenous political organizations began to form, and agitation was felt almost immediately.

On the whole, in the unsettled colonies where the white population was minimal (such as Nigeria), the handover of power was a matter of grooming a new generation of leadership to receive power. In colonies such as Kenya, Rhodesia, and the future Zimbabwe, where large and settled white populations existed, the situation was likely to be a great deal more complicated. What the nascent liberation movements lacked, however, was the authentic scope of a mass movement to challenge powerful white hegemony in these colonies, and this the whites handed to them over the question of land.

Hundreds of thousands of white British troops were leaving the armed services and departing a ruined Europe in droves for the colonies. To attract them, the individual colonial governments were offering generous land grants while pushing the indigenous black population off the land to make way. It was this issue, the theft of the land, that finally gave the liberation movements the manpower to mount mass action and then to form armies and fight wars. By the 1960s, the African liberation movement was well underway, and by the end of the 1970s, it was largely complete. The war cry of the revolution was *A Luta Continua* ("The struggle continues") and "One Man One Vote."

In 1953, the decision had been made within the central African colonies to federate the three British territories of Northern and Southern Rhodesia and Nyasaland. This was in order to try and find some safety in numbers. The British government was extremely reluctant to authorize anything along these lines, but nonetheless, under enormous pressure, it did so. There was, at the same time, huge pressure brought to bear against the British government to disallow this course of action, most notably from the domestic black nationalist movement, but also from the United Nations and newly independent nation-states worldwide.

Nonetheless, the Federation of Rhodesia and Nyasaland came into existence August 1, 1953. It was founded on a complicated constitutional framework that was designed to allow for a certain amount of black representation, but under rules that manifestly limited black progress. So unpopular was the move that any black involvement in it was regarded as collaborationist. The entire enterprise was boycotted by the substantive nationalist branches, with only the occasional moderate or traditional leader submitting to cooperation with the government.

The Central African Federation was the cause of widespread black protest and civil unrest, and although this subsided somewhat once it became de facto, resistance to it was ongoing. The main focus of objection was

Nyasaland, and in the end, it would be Nyasaland that would bring the edifice down.

The first British territory to gain independence was the Gold Coast, which passed from British to local rule on March 6, 1957, hard on the heels of the Suez Crisis. The nation-state thus created was Ghana, and Kwame Nkrumah was its first Prime Minister. The Gold Coast had always been a supremely pleasant posting for those foreign service types fortunate enough to have been dispatched there. It was never one of the settled colonies, so its expatriate European community was small, and it was not, in the end, a difficult process to divest it.

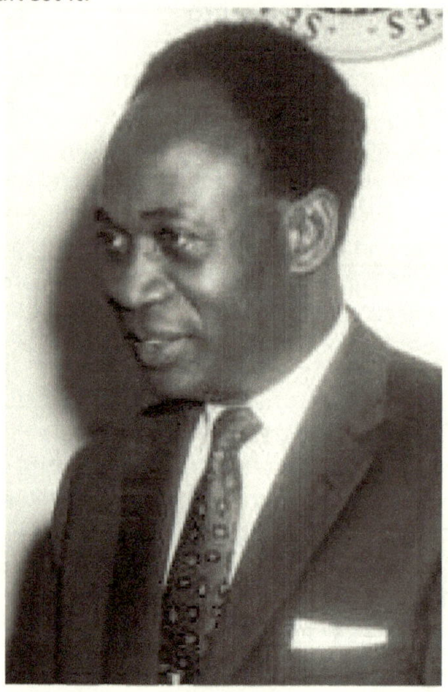

Nkrumah

Nkrumah seemed at times to be a rowdy fellow, overanxious for power and, once given power, apt to align his thinking east. He pictured himself as a prophet of African socialism, and as his familiarity with power began to get the better of him, he even dared to see himself as the leader of a united federation of Africa.

Regardless, Gold Coast independence was the starting pistol for the independence movement in the rest of British Africa. British West African territories left the fold soon afterward, with only Nigeria plunging almost immediately into a vicious separatist war that came to be known as the Biafran War and which was fought between 1967 and 1970.

In the crowd witnessing Kwame Nkrumah's inauguration was a 59-year old Nyasa doctor by the name of Hastings Banda. Banda was twice qualified, studying medicine first at the Meharry College in Tennessee and again at the University of Edinburgh, and in recent years he had established a busy general practice in North London. He was a physically unprepossessing man, habitually dressed in a dark, three-piece suit, a homburg hat, and a pair of dark sunglasses. But what he lacked in physical stature, he made up for in gumption. If Kwame Nkrumah had been a dream to the British Colonial Office, then Banda was about to become its nightmare.

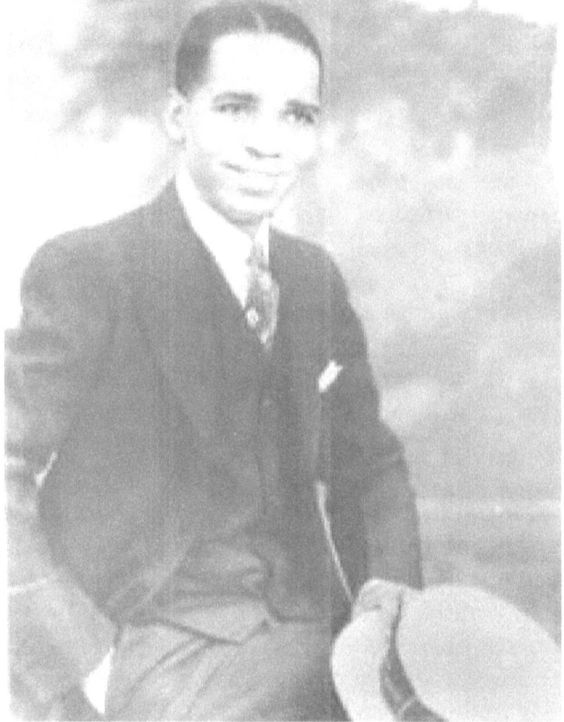

Banda

Nyasaland had, since its inception, been a protectorate characterized by a liberal and protective colonial administration and a politically alert native population. It was in the nature of the southern African economic dynamic at that time that labor was being drawn into the region from throughout the surrounding colonies. Most were being sucked into the emerging mining industry of South Africa and Rhodesia and into agricultural and industrial sectors all over the southern African region. In consequence, Nyasa political ideas were spreading along the arteries of migrant labor and inspiring movement across the subcontinent. There was, therefore, a certain inevitability about the fact that Nyasaland would prove to be the test case for southern African independence.

Banda was pulled into the vortex of this, not because of his brilliance, but because of the impoverishment of the political pool. He was educated, he was articulate, he was of the generation, and he was ambitious. The Nyasaland African Congress evolved, as did similar African nationalist political parties in most British territories, from Christian/missionary organizations through the gamut of vigilance societies, social clubs, debating groups, action groups, and finally fully fledged political parties. Nyasaland Congress, however, unlike most, was given a largely free reign by a benign colonial administration to form and campaign within the colony as it chose. Its mood, therefore, was aggressive, and its agenda was the dissolution of the Central African Federation and a prompt grant of independence from the Crown. All that it lacked was a charismatic leader.

In July 1958, Banda appeared in the colony, assuming leadership of Congress and launching immediately into an abrasive and violent campaign of civil disobedience. It is interesting that he had been out of the country for so long that he had forgotten his native language, and so his speeches were translated from English by an interpreter. On the surface, they seemed moderate and restrained, but when translated into idiomatic Chewa, they became incendiary and voluble, urging action and firing the passions of a nation aroused.

The anxiety in white society that this provoked tended not to be in Nyasaland itself but in Southern Rhodesia mainly, where a similarly configured Congress party was finding its feet and where the settler population had the most to lose. Banda was courting arrest, and the more reluctant the office of the local governor was to issue a warrant of arrest, the more provocative became his actions. Banda's favorite remark during this wave of positive action was, "When the British start arresting, full independence is around the corner."

On March 3, 1959, a state of emergency was finally declared, and federal troops moved in to quell the disturbances. Banda was arrested and detained as he hoped, and quite as he had expected, his new role as a prisoner of conscience propelled his profile and the freedom campaign to the forefront of the imperial debate. A peremptory state of emergency was declared soon afterward in Southern Rhodesia, where the leading nationalists were rounded up and detained just to subdue their ability to add to the general mayhem.

Meanwhile, and notwithstanding a great deal of hand-wringing and pleading from the various colonial administrations, the British government, through its usual device of a commission of inquiry, arrived at the conclusion that the Federation was no longer tenable. Moreover, succession by Nyasaland, bearing in mind the political realities of the age, would be an inevitable precursor to independence. And if Nyasaland seceded, then so would Northern Rhodesia, which was already starting to ramp up its own campaign of positive action in expectation of a similar imperial capitulation. Thereafter, quite frankly, what would be the point of a federation with one member?

And so it was that on December 31, 1963, after 10 years of existence, the controversial Federation of Rhodesia and Nyasaland was dissolved. On July 6, 1964, Nyasaland was granted independence from the British crown, marking the birth of the nation-state of Malawi. Three months later, Northern Rhodesia followed suit, entering the world stage as the Republic of Zambia, led by the affable and charismatic Kenneth Kaunda.

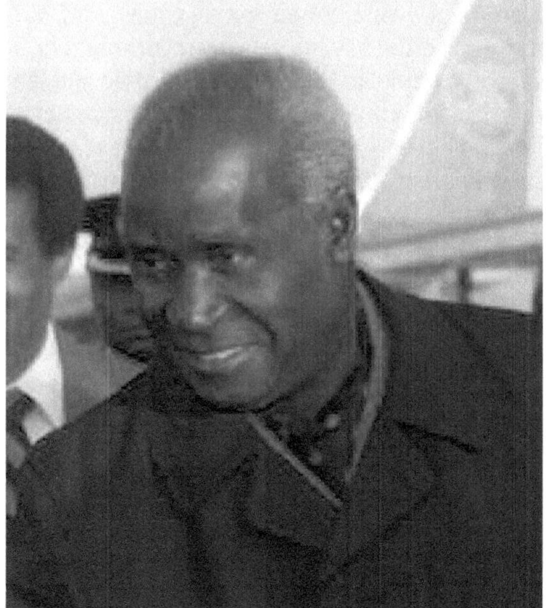

Kaunda

As this indicated, African liberation movements often devolved into political unrest and civil wars, and the collapse of communism in 1989 and the end of the Cold War brought about a great many changes across continent. Most importantly, it marked the end of Cold War patronage that had supported and sustained so much negative and destructive leadership in Africa. A great many regimes toppled in the aftermath of this, and Africa was to a large degree cleansed by it. It also meant the end of white South African control of South West Africa and the beginning of the end of apartheid.

The end of the Cold War also brought about the most disastrous episode of all. Somalia was the only territory subject to colonization that mounted a successful resistance. The Italians had an interest in the region as their contribution to the great civilizing mission in Africa, but the British were also interested in it for its strategic relevance, as was the independent kingdom of Ethiopia. It took a 20-year military campaign to finally subjugate the territory, and even then, pacification was only partial.

During World War II, the Italians took control of Ethiopia and Somalia in their entirety, and one of the early campaigns fought was that to liberate it. Ethiopia was returned to its monarchy, and after the war, the Italians were granted a United Nations mandate to govern southern Somalia, while the British retained British Somalia, congruent with modern-day Somaliland.

Somalia was granted independence in 1960, and the country was unified. Indigenous government over a united Somalia, however, was almost within itself an oxymoron. Traditionally, no central government or unified control had ever taken root in Somalia. The nomadic lifestyle and individualistic mindset characteristic of ethnic Somali clansmen tended to preclude it, while historic attrition over water, livestock, and other resources further complicated a bewildering ebb and flow of loyalties, enmities, alliances, and conflicts. The inevitable conclusion was that national unity was quickly subverted to narrow clan interests. A plethora of competing political parties and the selective distribution of patronage based on clan and family became the pattern leading up to a military coup mounted in October 1969, transfering power from civilian to military leadership. The new government, Scientific Socialist in its stated ideological alignment, was headed by army commander Major General Mohamed Siad Barre.

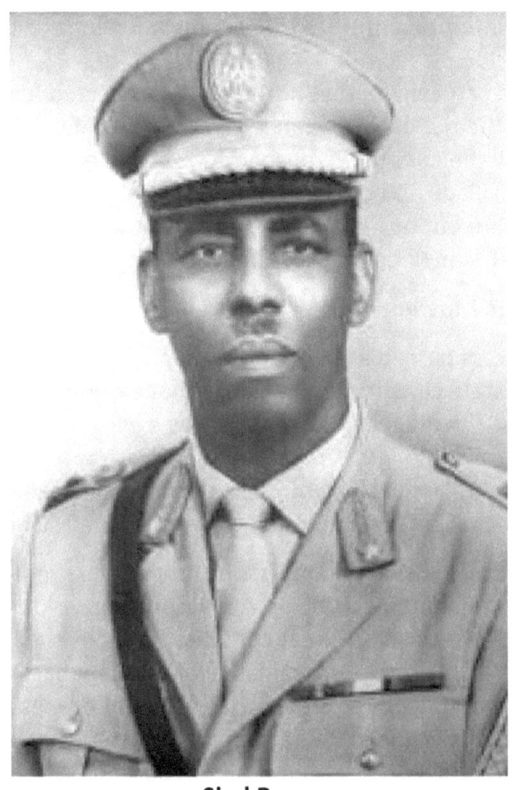

Siad Barre

Siad Barre, a well-adjusted Machiavellian, held power in a regime characterized by repression, military ambition, and greed that could claim but one achievement: its ability, albeit nominally, to govern. Siad Barre, however, was ousted in 1991 as a coalition of various clans converged to achieve this limited objective before fracturing immediately thereafter into the preferred polarity of warlords, shifting clan alliances, and the rotating domination of the country by one group or another.

In 1992, the United States Marine Corps landed on the beaches of Mogadishu in an operation intended to separate the warring factions in order that food distribution might be undertaken by various aid agencies. U.S. troops were applauded as they arrived in the city, but less than two years later, that same population was filmed dragging the bodies of U.S. troops through the streets of Mogadishu, kicking and spitting on them in the aftermath of the famed Blackhawk Down incident. U.S. troops were soon withdrawn, and the episode contributed directly to the unwillingness of

President Bill Clinton to authorize U.S. action in Rwanda as the events of the Rwandan Genocide played out.

Somalia proved an enigma that no Western-concocted formula could heal, and in the end, the nation was abandoned to its own fate. That fate has tended to follow the continuum of shackled central government and a nation run on a village and clan level. Innovations have been attempted and might yet succeed, but one is certainly left with the impression that this quintessential African dilemma will remain one for some time to come.

The Civil Rights Movement

In 1867, Congress passed a law that required all the Confederate states to include in their state constitutions a clause that extended the vote to their black minorities. The main engine for this was a wing of the Republicancontrolled Congress regarded as radical for its strong position on this and other liberal issues. The motion was not universally popular, and as history would reveal, an enormous controversy proved to be the result.

Nonetheless, there was irony in this, because even as most of the Southern states implemented universal male suffrage, older voting laws remained in effect in the North that continued to deny the black man the vote. At the same time, the predominance of the Republican Party in the North – at the time the liberal/progressive wing of Congress – saw its share of the vote steadily decline in the face of the more conservative and restrictive Democratic Party, at that time the party of the South. The Republican social agenda was obviously not universally popular in the North, and in an effort to balance things out more in the Republicans' favor, it was suggested that extending suffrage to male blacks in the North would bring more Republican voters out.

This was still easier said than done. Notwithstanding the dynamics of the Civil War, voting rights for black men in the North remained a deeply unpopular idea, and in fact a number of Northern states had recently voted against black suffrage. The change came in 1868 when the Republican Party held its presidential nominating convention in Chicago, selecting as their candidate the renowned Civil War hero Ulysses S. Grant. While continuing to hold that black male suffrage would be a requirement in the South, in the Republican stronghold of the North, the matter was left open. Grant emerged victorious in the election of that year with such a slim majority that it became clear that the party could not hope to survive without the black vote.

This, then, was the background to the Fifteenth Amendment. Deliberations began during the 1869 Congressional session, and after numerous versions of the proposed amendment were presented and rejected, a compromise was eventually agreed that was vaguely enough worded to cove the voting rights of black men with specific mention. Section 1 of it read simply, "The right of citizens of the United States to vote shall not be denied or abridged by the United States or by any State on account of race, color, or previous condition of servitude."

This won the required two-thirds majority in Congress, after which 28 states in the Union were required to ratify it. In 11 Southern states, the matter already existed under the law, so just 17 other states were required to support the amendment for it to become Federal law. Nine of these states already allowed black men to vote, so the decision really rested on the swing of only eight states.

Needless to say, the Democratic Party realized that this was a fight for its political survival. The ratification of the Fifteenth Amendment would automatically establish 170,000 loyal black Republican voters throughout the North and West, and so the party fought a spirited campaign against the amendment, claiming in essence that it interfered with the rights of the individual states to run their own elections. Numerous spurious arguments were lodged in favor of the independence of individual states in this matter, among them the high rates of illiteracy among blacks, their political immaturity, and the likelihood of them being swayed by false promises and bribery.

For their part, the Republicans steadily fought, state by state, clinching the argument by bringing Georgia, the last and most determinedly racist state, on board. The Fifteenth Amendment was officially proclaimed part of the Constitution of the United States on March 30, 1870, prompting celebrations in some states and ominous silence in others. As 10,000 people marched through the streets of Baltimore, Frederick Douglass, in a speech delivered on May 5, 1870, proclaimed, "What a country – fortunate in its institutions, in its 15th Amendment, in its future."

Lofty words aside, Douglass likely understood there was a lot of obstacles to still overcome. In the South, a negative reaction was almost immediate. The Ku Klux Klan and various other violent racist organizations began an intense campaign to intimidate blacks out of voting by burning their churches, schools, and homes, and frequently resorting to extrajudicial killings. All the while, under federal protection, blacks voted, won elected offices, and served on juries, and while lynchings, arson, and violence went on largely unchecked, there was a sense of optimism that things would work out.

Then, in 1876, things changed. In the election of that year, the electoral votes were disputed, and the Republicans ultimately struck a deal with the Southern Democrats. In exchange for Southern recognition and support for the election of Republican presidential candidate Rutherford B. Hayes, the Republicans undertook to remove all troops from the South, effectively removing federal protection of the exercise of the black franchise. It was both a practical and symbolic move, and almost overnight, the black community of the South found itself at the mercy of a largely belligerent and racist white population.

Civil War historian James McPherson noted that the end of Reconstruction ultimately was brought about by the "wavering commitment" of Northern Republicans. Due in part to Southern castigation of Reconstruction, Northern society had become disillusioned with carpetbaggers and was not committed to black rights. The war's "revolutionary achievements" had thus been based more on anti-Southern motivation than pro-black sentiment. To "emancipationist" writers, most notably Frederick Douglass and W.E.B. DuBois, "Reconstruction required a full accounting of the past," an accounting that was not coming in the foreseeable future. Though they appealed to people to remember the necessity of Reconstruction for black Americans, their vision would be obscured in the North out of political expediency.

It would take another 80 years before historians started to challenge the view of Reconstruction as being a harsh and detrimental occupation of the South. Taking Southern institutions like Jim Crow and the Ku Klux Klan into account, Reconstruction historians since the 1960s have viewed Republican Reconstruction in a considerably more positive light. Directly answering some of the commonly held views of Reconstruction, McPherson argued that "the postwar era...affected the South as it affected the rest of the country." Southerners had cast a pall over "Negro Rule" Reconstruction in their writings and memory, despite the fact that blacks never held more than 20% of the political offices in the South.

The end of Reconstruction brought about the Jim Crow South in short order. Jim Crow was a theater persona created by the American actor and playwright Thomas D. Rice, who wrote the character and performed him in blackface makeup, using black vernacular speech and song and dance. The character was based on folk tales describing a lovable trickster with the name Jim Crow. The term at the time was not pejorative, and it was widely viewed as a trope that bridged different cultures, generating greater awareness and sympathy for black culture. How it came to be associated with a raft of discriminatory laws in the South that followed Reconstruction is not entirely known, but the term very quickly acquired a darker meaning as the gains of Reconstruction were steadily rolled back.

Discretionary laws found expression on state statutes all across the South, especially as economic depression gripped the region in the 1890s. Competition for scarce jobs made social and economic discrimination against blacks extremely attractive. It became fashionable for politicians to abuse blacks for the sake of winning white votes, while the myth of black criminality and sexual violence fueled an increasingly violent response.

In 1890, the Louisiana state assembly, notwithstanding having six elected black members, passed a law prohibiting white and black people from traveling on the same bus. A challenge was mounted that eventually was heard by the Supreme Court in the 1896 landmark case *Plessy v. Ferguson*. The Supreme Court ultimately upheld the Louisiana law, creating the infamous doctrine of "separate but equal."

This, in and of itself, did not necessarily interfere with the provision of the Fifteenth Amendment, but multiple obstacles and restrictions were placed in the paths of black access to the vote. This was codified in 1898 with the upholding by the Supreme Court of a Mississippi law requiring a literacy test and proof of payment of a poll tax before an adult male of any color would be permitted to vote. The requirement was not deemed unconstitutional or discriminatory, and it drastically increased the number of disenfranchised blacks, for the poll tax was required to be paid retroactively, while a grandfather clause had the effect of excepting whites, but not blacks.

From that point on, Jim Crow laws expanded rapidly in all of the Southern states, touching every aspect of life, and while the Supreme Court ruling of 1896 opened the way for the principle of "separate but equal," the practical effect of most Jim Crow laws was simply to enforce segregation. Prisons, hospitals, schools and universities were segregated. While in the South much of this was a matter of law, in other cities in the United States – as far afield as New York, Chicago and Los Angeles – discrimination also touched every aspect of life. As a result, even as the rights of minorities to vote were never technically infringed upon in words by the Jim Crow laws, social conditions were such that any black person in virtually any Southern state who sought to exercise his right to vote ran the very real risk of intimidation, violence, and lynching. Democrats held a firm grip on power in the South, and the situation perpetuated itself throughout the first half of the 20th century until the advent of the Civil Rights Movement in the 1950s helped bring about landmark legislation in 1964 and 1965.

The federal legislation, which made illegal any kind of discrimination in voting, came during the height of the Civil Rights Movement and was signed into law by President Lyndon B. Johnson. The law was designed to enforce the voting rights guaranteed under the Fifteenth Amendment, securing the right to vote for all racial minorities. According to a publication circulated by the Department of Justice, the Voting Rights Act of 1965 is considered the most effective piece of federal civil rights legislation ever enacted in the country.

Conclusion

The 1960s was the decade that saw the culmination of both the Civil Rights
Movement in the United States and the beginning of the African Liberation Movement. Both were watershed moments in the journey towards full emancipation and fair voting rights. By the end of the 1960s, Africa – with the exception of southern Africa – was entering an era of liberation. The 1970s would be the period of war in southern Africa as the Portuguese colonies of Angola and Mozambique were liberated, and in 1980, Zimbabwe. South Africa would prove to be a somewhat tougher nut to crack, but the eventual collapse of the Soviet Union and the rearrangement of the world order eventually brought the monumental edifice of white rule in South

Africa down. When Nelson Mandela walked free in February 1990, African liberation could finally be said to be complete.

The African experience under liberation was mixed to say the very least. A bitter joke circulated as Africa settled into its first phase of liberation: "One Man One Vote Once." Almost without exception, liberated African governments fell to military rule or kleptocratic dictatorships under conditions of one party rule. The rationale behind much of this was the inability of Africa to function as a modern democracy when nations defined by arbitrary colonial borders contained mutually antagonistic tribes. While in every respect this ideology was used to perpetuate dictatorships and military governments, some truth certainly lay in the assertion that Africans would always vote along tribal lines, and that numerically dominant tribes would always rule by force of numbers. It was generally claimed that democracy was ill-suited to the African model and that benign dictatorship and "bigman" politics suited the continent better.

Many of these dictatorships survived thanks to Cold War patronage, and the notion of democracy withered to the point where many governments barely went to the effort to hold elections. The end of the Cold War shifted the balance considerably, and as old regimes fell like dominoes, for the first time, the shoots of authentic democracy took root.

democracy was ill-suited to the African model and that benign dictatorship and "bigman" politics suited the continent better.

Many of these dictatorships survived thanks to Cold War patronage, and the notion of democracy withered to the point where many governments barely went to the effort to hold elections. The end of the Cold War shifted the balance considerably, and as old regimes fell like dominoes, for the first time, the shoots of authentic democracy took root.

www.ingramcontent.com/pod-product-compliance
Lightning Source LLC
Chambersburg PA
CBHW021355160726
47994CB00007B/2958